40 INSPIRATIONAL

BIBLE VERSES

Copyright © 2023 Brad Chambers
ISBN# 9798385637966

So whether you eat or drink or whatever you do, do it all for the glory of God

1 Corinthians 10:31

Therefore, my dear brothers and sisters, stand firm. Let nothing move you. Always give yourselves fully to the work of the Lord, because you know that your labor in the Lord is not in vain.

1 Corinthians 15:58

We love because he first loved us.

1 John 4:19

"My grace is sufficient for you, for my power is made perfect in weakness"

2 Corinthians 12:9

Let your roots grow down into him, and let your lives be built on him. Then your faith will grow strong in the truth you were taught, and you will overflow with thankfulness.

Colossians 2:7

And be kind to one another, tenderhearted, forgiving one another, even as God in Christ forgave you.

Ephesians 4:32

The Lord shall fight for you, and ye shall hold your peace.

Exodus 14:14

So then faith cometh by hearing, and hearing by the word of God

Romans 10:17

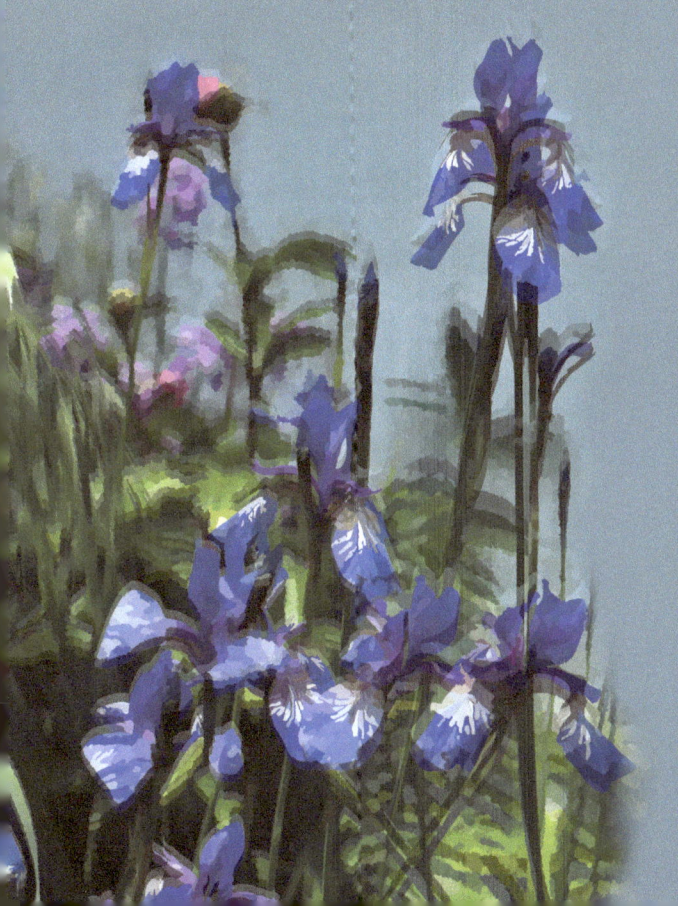

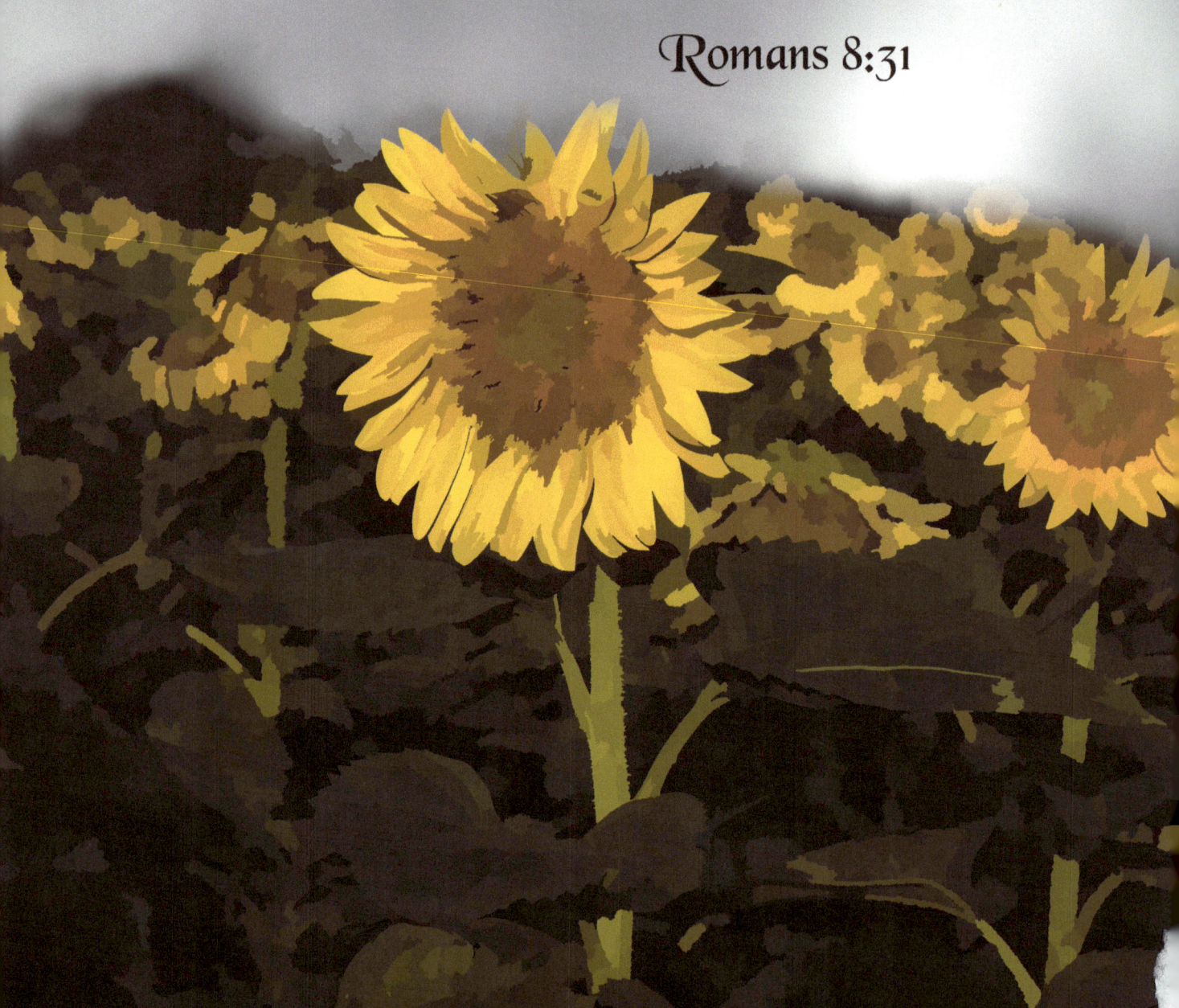

So do not fear, for I am with you;
do not be dismayed, for I am your God.
I will strengthen you and help you;
I will uphold you with my righteous right hand.

Isaiah 41:10

For ye shall go out with joy,

And be led forth with peace:

The mountains and the hills

shall break forth before

you into singing,

And all the trees of the field

shall clap their hands.

Isaiah 55:12

Jabez cried out to the God of Israel, "Oh, that you would bless me and enlarge my territory! Let your hand be with me, and keep me from harm so that I will be free from pain." And God granted his request.

Before I formed you in the womb I knew you, before you were born I set you apart

Jeremiah 1:5

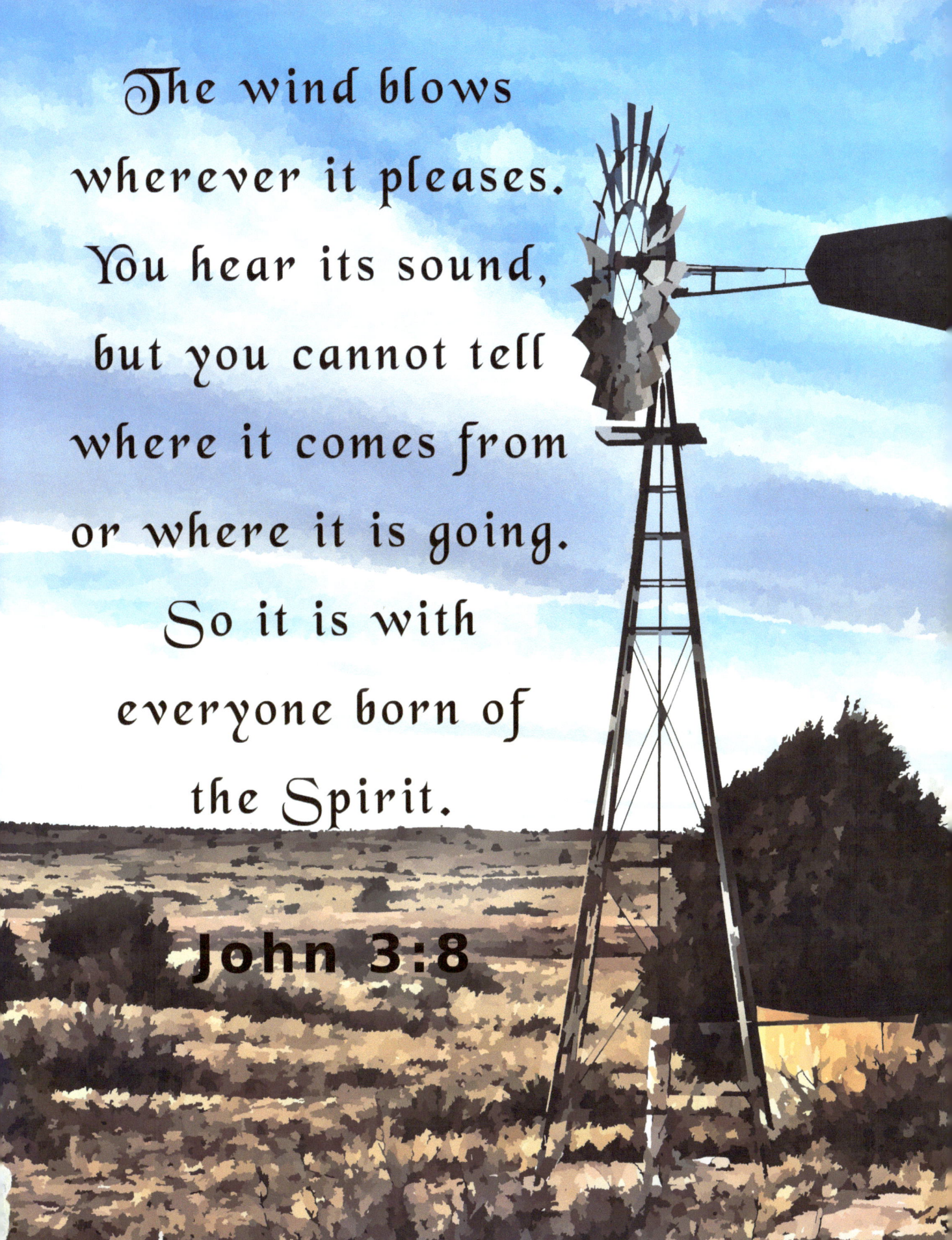

For God so loved the world, that he gave his only begotten Son, that whosoever believeth in him should not perish, but have everlasting life.

John 3:16

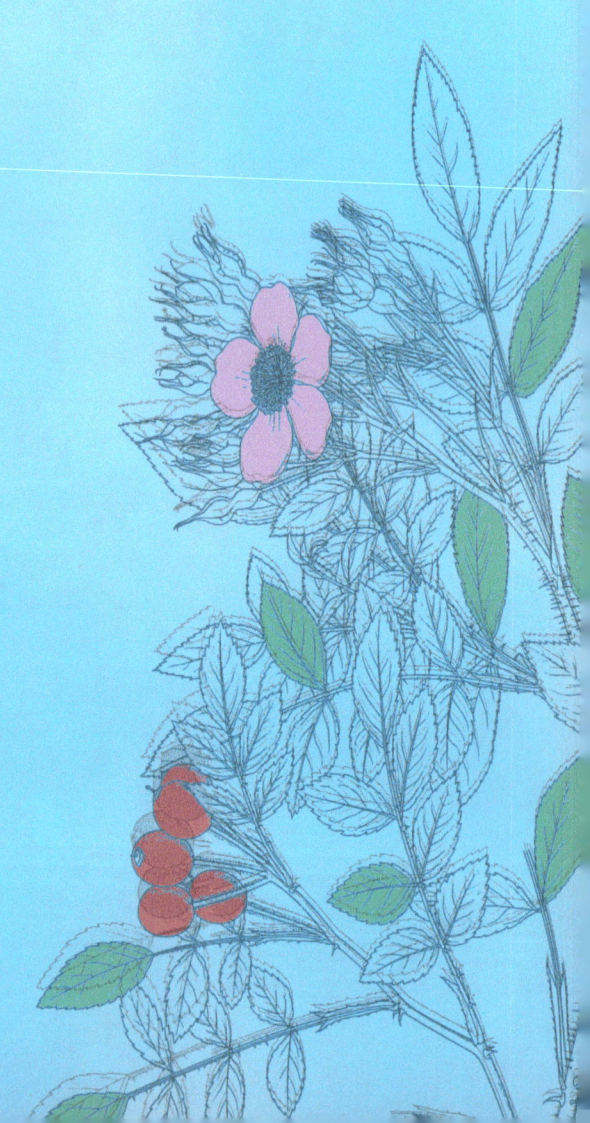

I have come that they may have life; and that they may have it more abundantly.

John 10:10

Be strong and courageous. Do not be afraid; do not be discouraged, for the Lord your God will be with you wherever you go.

Joshua 1:9

Yet this I call to mind and therefore I have hope: Because of the Lord's great love we are not consumed, for his compassions never fail. They are new every morning; great is your faithfulness.

Lamentations 3:21-23

May the Lord of peace himself give you peace at all times in every way.

2 Thessalonians 3:16

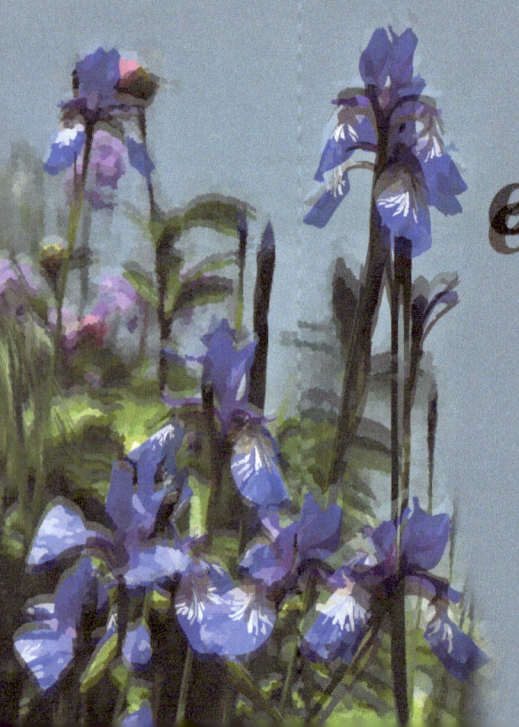
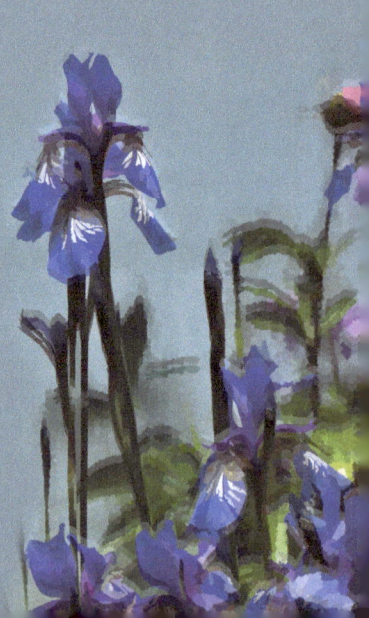

But seek first the kingdom of God and His righteousness, and all these things shall be added to you.

Mathew 6:33

Come unto me, all ye that labour and are heavy laden, and I will give you rest.

Mathew 11:28

For with God nothing shall be impossible

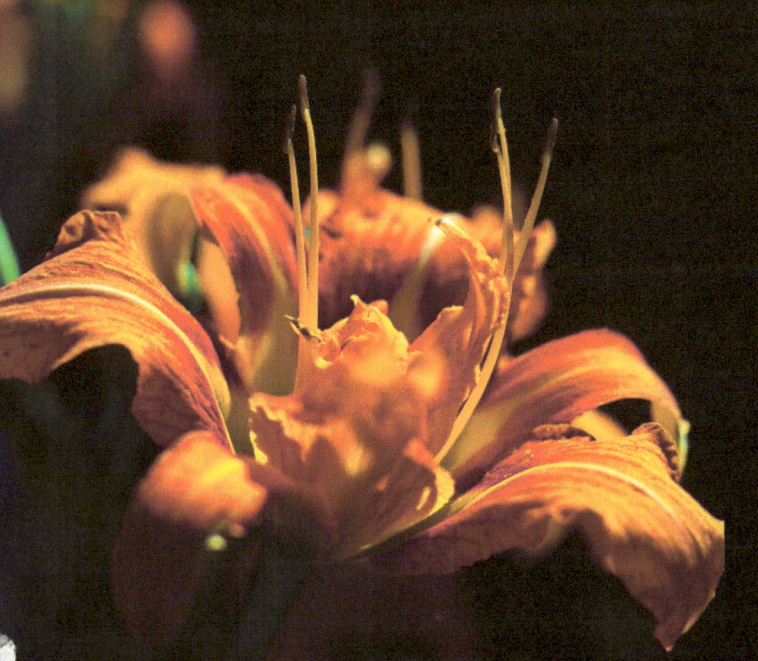

Luke 1:37

And the peace of God, which surpasses all understanding, will guard your hearts and minds through Christ Jesus.

Philippians 4:7

Trust in the Lord with all your heart and lean not on your own understanding; in all your ways submit to him, and he will make your paths straight

Proverbs 3:5-6

Above all else, guard your heart, for everything you do flows from it.

Proverbs 4:23

Commit to the LORD whatever you do, and He will establish your plans.

Proverbs 16:3

She opens her mouth with wisdom, and the teaching of kindness is on her tongue.

Proverbs 31:26

In peace I will lie down and sleep, for you alone, Lord, make me dwell in safety.

Psalm 4:8

Psalm 16:8

I have set the Lord always before me; because He is at my right hand, I shall not be shaken.

I remain confident in this: I will see the goodness of the Lord in the land of the living

Psalm 27:13

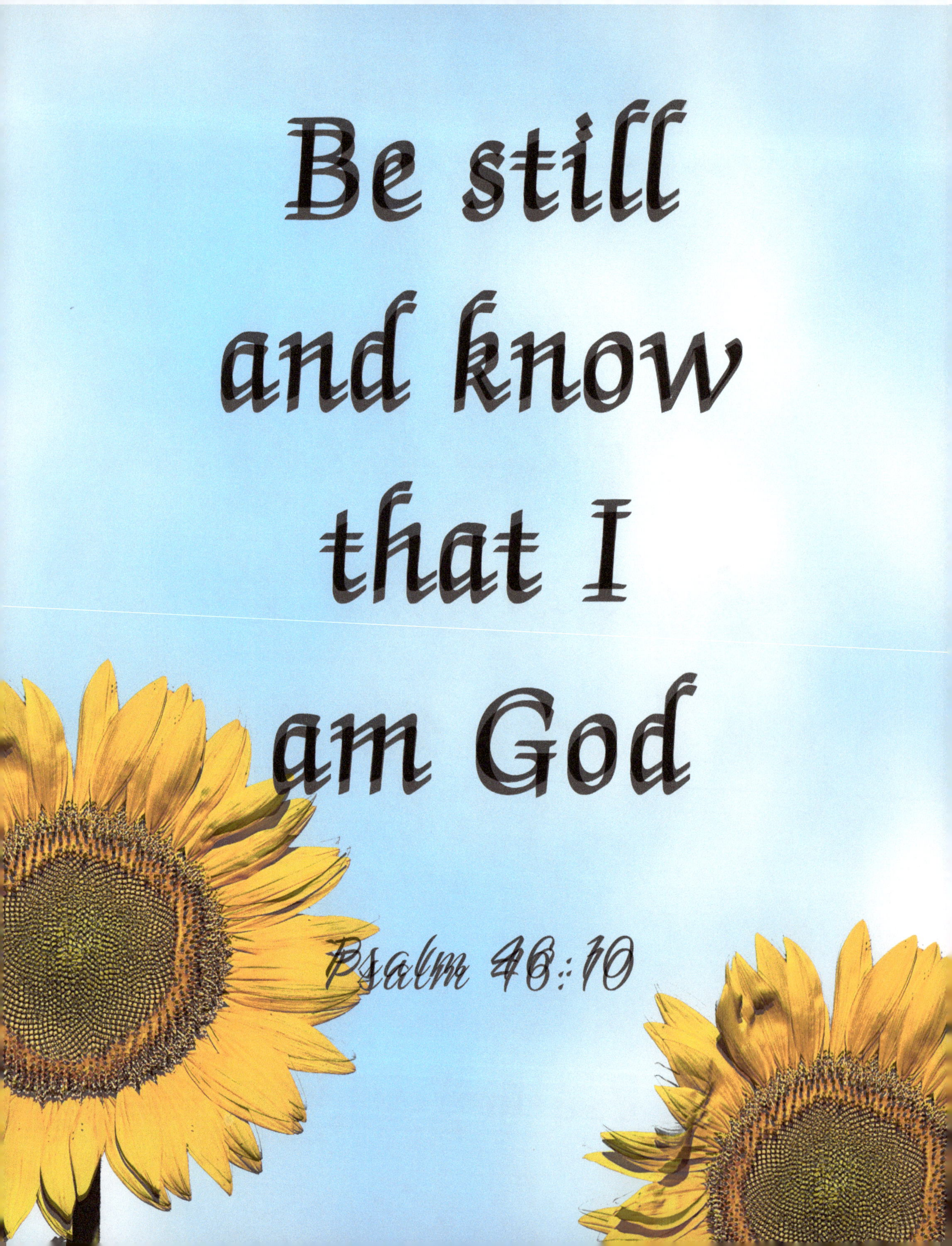

Be still and know that I am God

Psalm 46:10

Psalm 61:2

From the end of the earth I will cry to You; When my heart is overwhelmed; Lead me to the rock that is higher than I.

My flesh and my heart may fail, but God is the strength of my heart and my portion forever.

Psalm 73:26

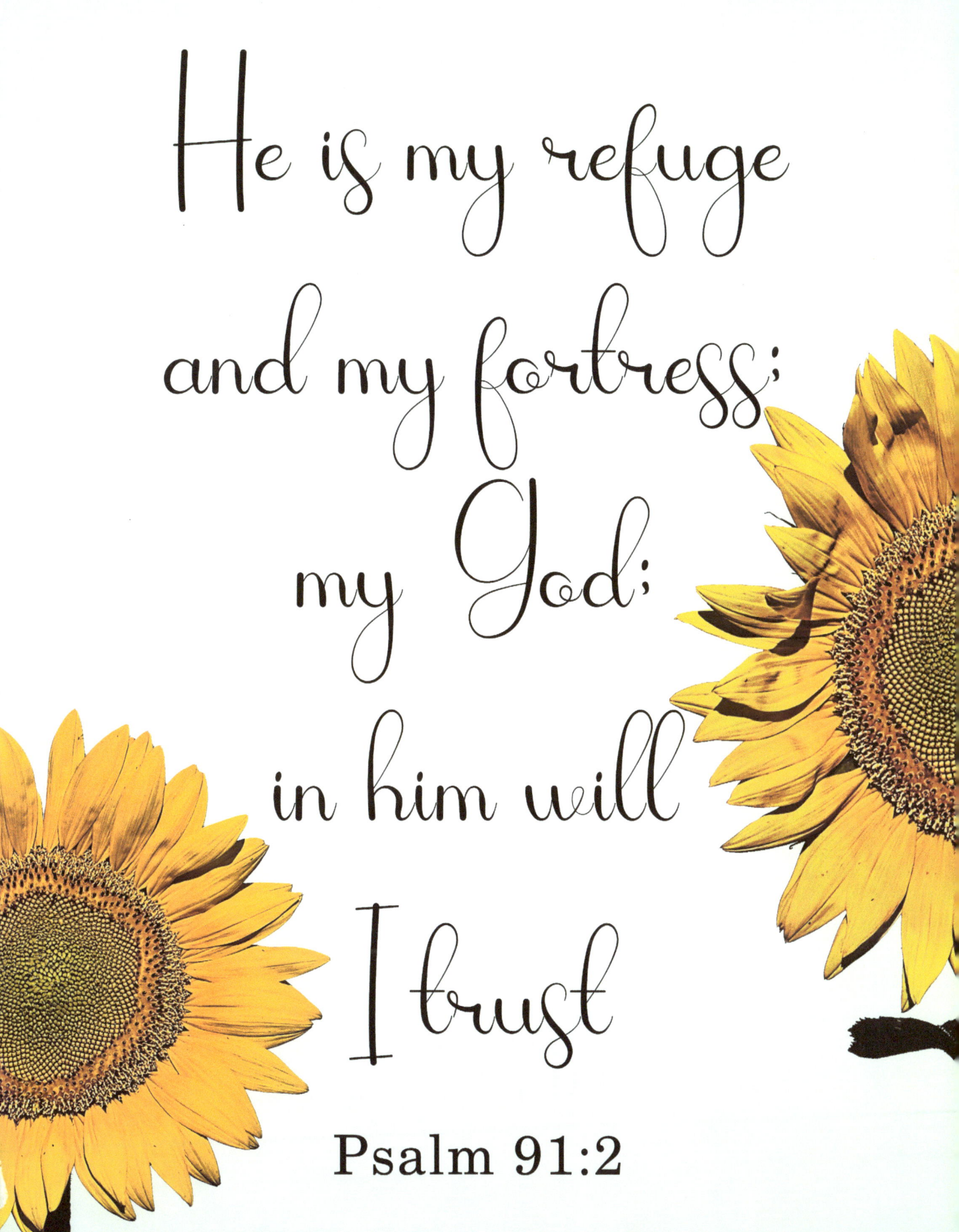

This is the day which the LORD hath made; we will rejoice and be glad in it.

Psalm 118:24

I will lift up mine eyes unto the hills, from whence cometh my help. My help cometh from the Lord, which made heaven and earth.

Psalm 121:1-2

Let the morning bring me word of your unfailing love, for I have put my trust in you. Show me the way I should go, for to you I entrust my life.

Psalm 143:8

And we know that in all things

God works for the good

of those who love him,

who have been called

according to his purpose

Romans 8:28

And be not conformed to this world: but be ye transformed by the renewing of your mind, that ye may prove what is that good, and acceptable, and perfect, will of God.

Romans 12:2

May the God of hope fill you with all joy and peace as you trust in him, so that you may overflow with hope by the power of the Holy Spirit.

Romans 15:13

The Lord bless you and keep you; the Lord make his face shine on you and be gracious to you; the Lord turn his face toward you and give you peace.

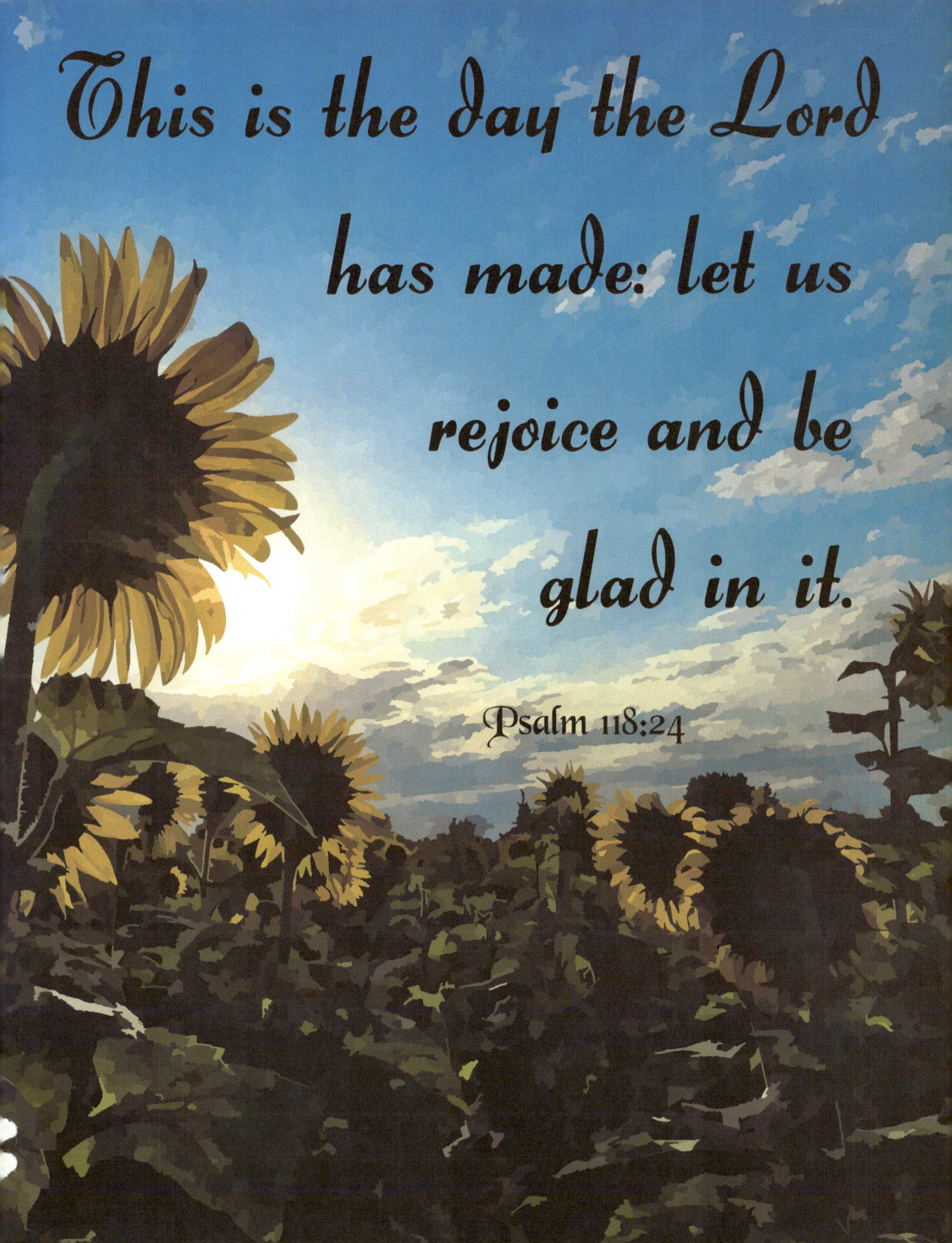